Your Amazing Body

Mouth

by Imogen Kingsley

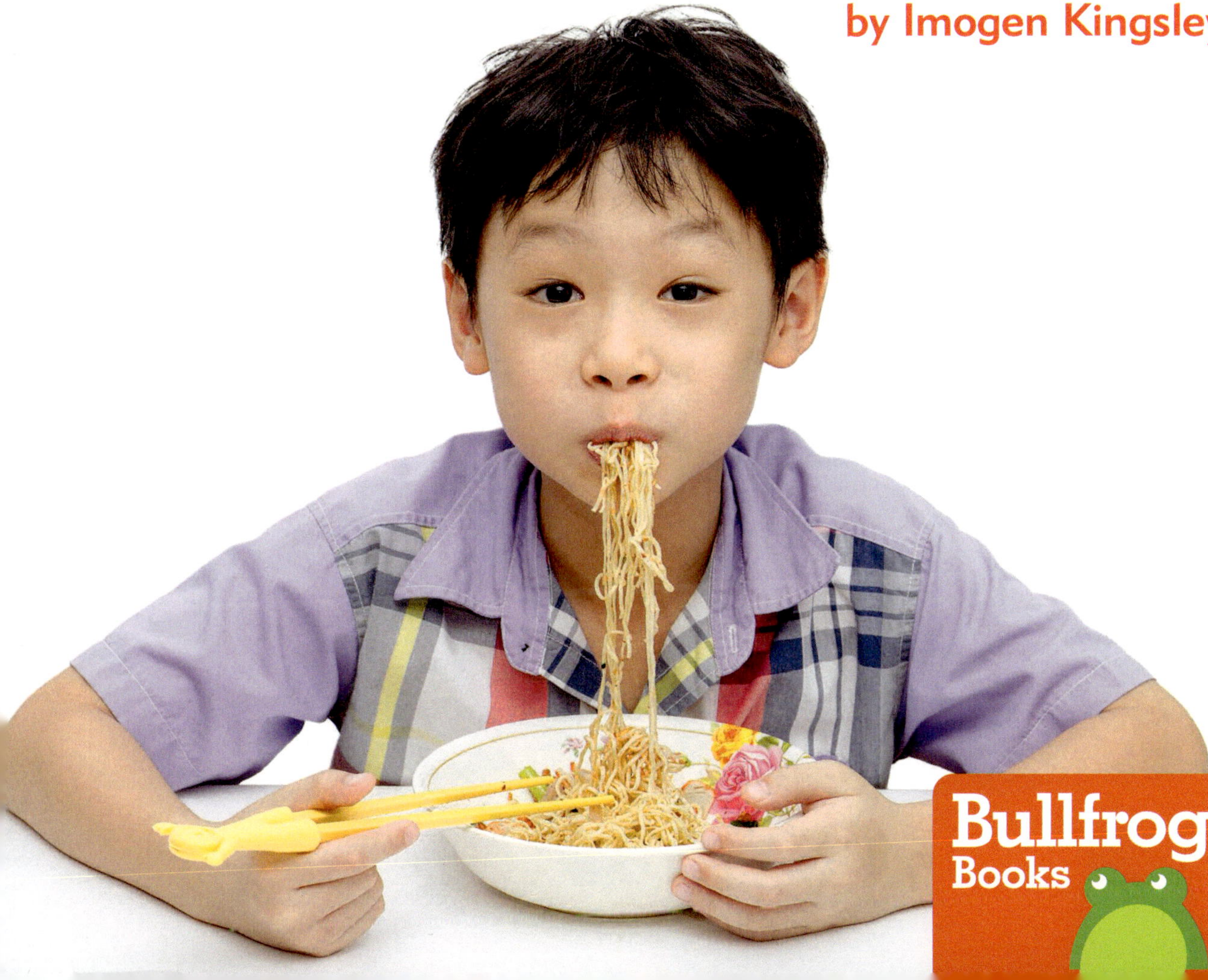

Bullfrog Books

Ideas for Parents and Teachers

Bullfrog Books let children practice reading informational text at the earliest reading levels. Repetition, familiar words, and photo labels support early readers.

Before Reading

- Discuss the cover photo. What does it tell them?
- Look at the picture glossary together. Read and discuss the words.

Read the Book

- "Walk" through the book and look at the photos. Let the child ask questions. Point out the photo labels.
- Read the book to the child, or have him or her read independently.

After Reading

- Prompt the child to think more. Ask: Think of all the different flavors your tongue can identify. If you wanted to eat something bitter, what would you choose? How about salty? Or sweet?

Bullfrog Books are published by Jump!
5357 Penn Avenue South
Minneapolis, MN 55419
www.jumplibrary.com

Library of Congress Cataloging-in-Publication Data

Names: Kingsley, Imogen, author.
Title: Mouth / by Imogen Kingsley.
Description: Minneapolis, MN: Jump!, Inc., [2017]
Series: Your amazing body
"Bullfrog Books are published by Jump!"
Audience: Ages 5–8. Audience: K to grade 3.
Includes index.
Identifiers: LCCN 2016051698 (print)
LCCN 2016051837 (ebook)
ISBN 9781620316870 (hardcover: alk. paper)
ISBN 9781620317402 (pbk.)
ISBN 9781624965647 (ebook)
Subjects: LCSH: Mouth—Juvenile literature.
Anatomy—Juvenile literature.
Classification: LCC QM306 .K534 2017 (print)
LCC QM306 (ebook) | DDC 612.3/1—dc23
LC record available at https://lccn.loc.gov/2016051698

Editor: Jenny Fretland VanVoorst
Book Designer: Molly Ballanger
Photo Researcher: Molly Ballanger

Photo Credits: Alamy: Big Cheese Photo, 5. Getty: KidStock, 6–7. iStock: JodiJacobson, cover; Neustockimages, 14–15, kgfoto, 16; Mr_Khan, 18–19; kali9, 20–21. Shutterstock: all_about_people, 1, 8–9; michaeljung, 3; hanapon1002, 4; MAHATHIR MOHD YASIN, 10; ESB Professional, 11; BLUR LIFE 1975, 12–13; Sergiy Bykhunenko, 12–13; GongTo, 14–15; Marcos Mesa Sam Wordley, 17; 7th Son Studio, 18–19; Alila Medical Media, 22; Nathalie Speliers Ufermann, 22; DM7, 23bl; Asier Romero, 24.

Printed in the United States of America at Corporate Graphics in North Mankato, Minnesota.

Table of Contents

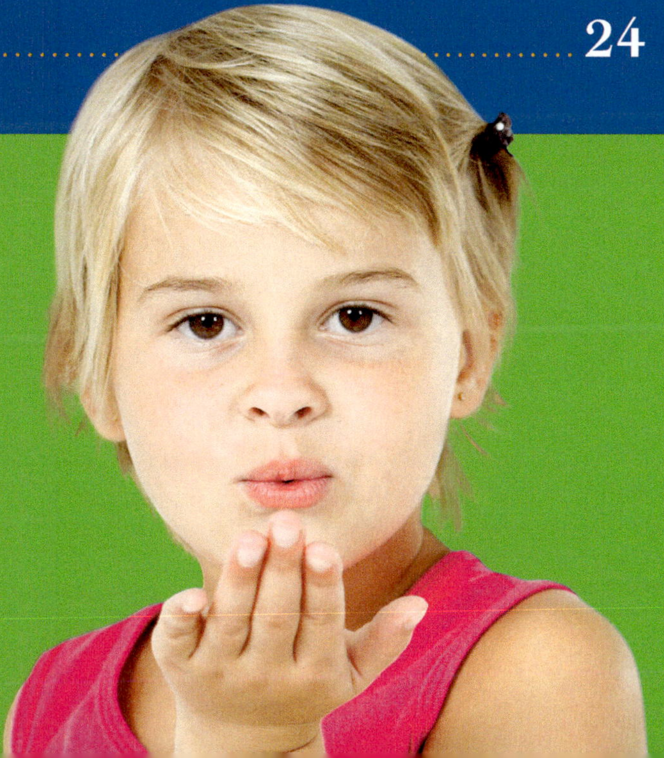

Open Wide!

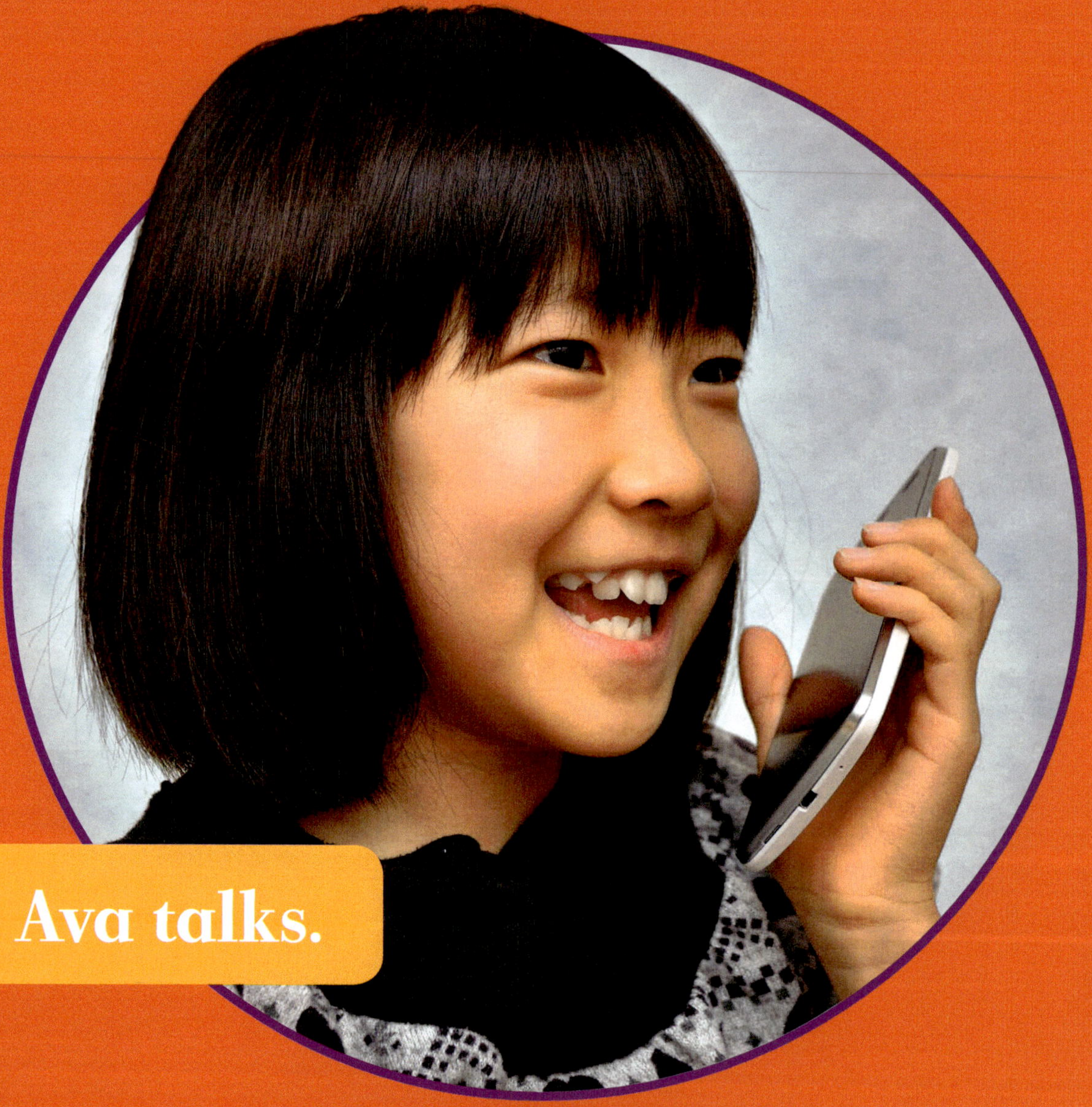

Ava talks.

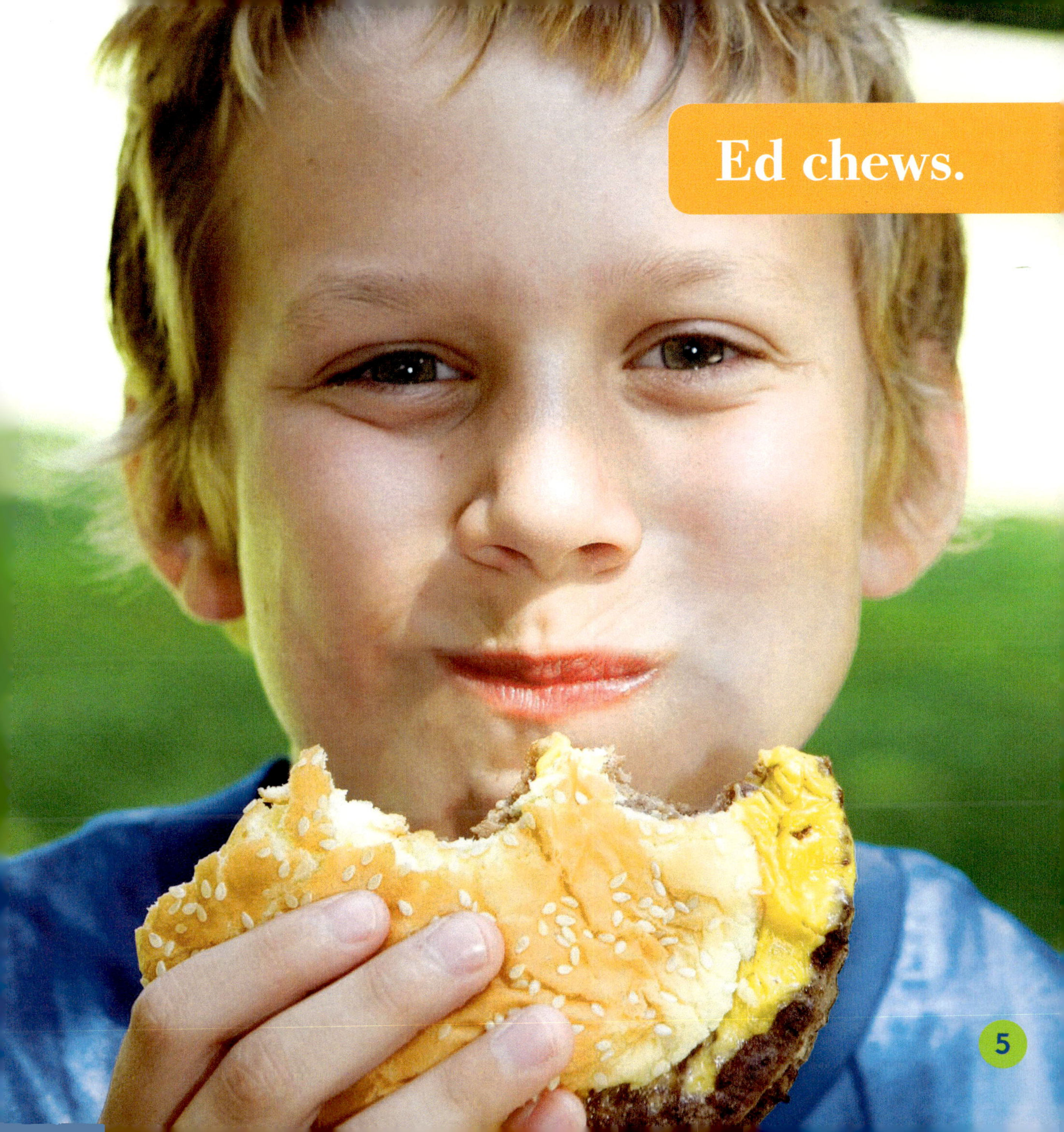

Ed chews.

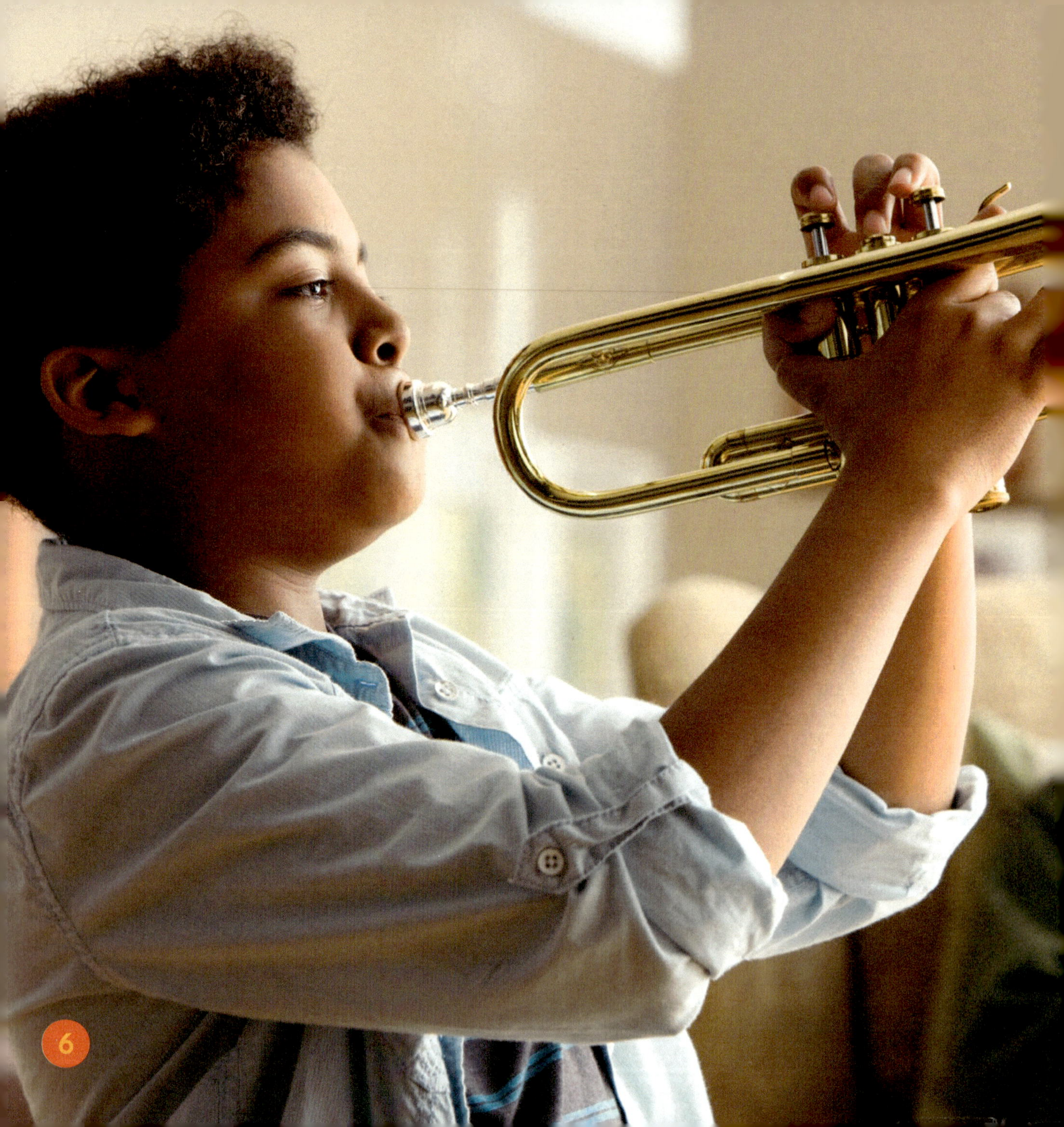

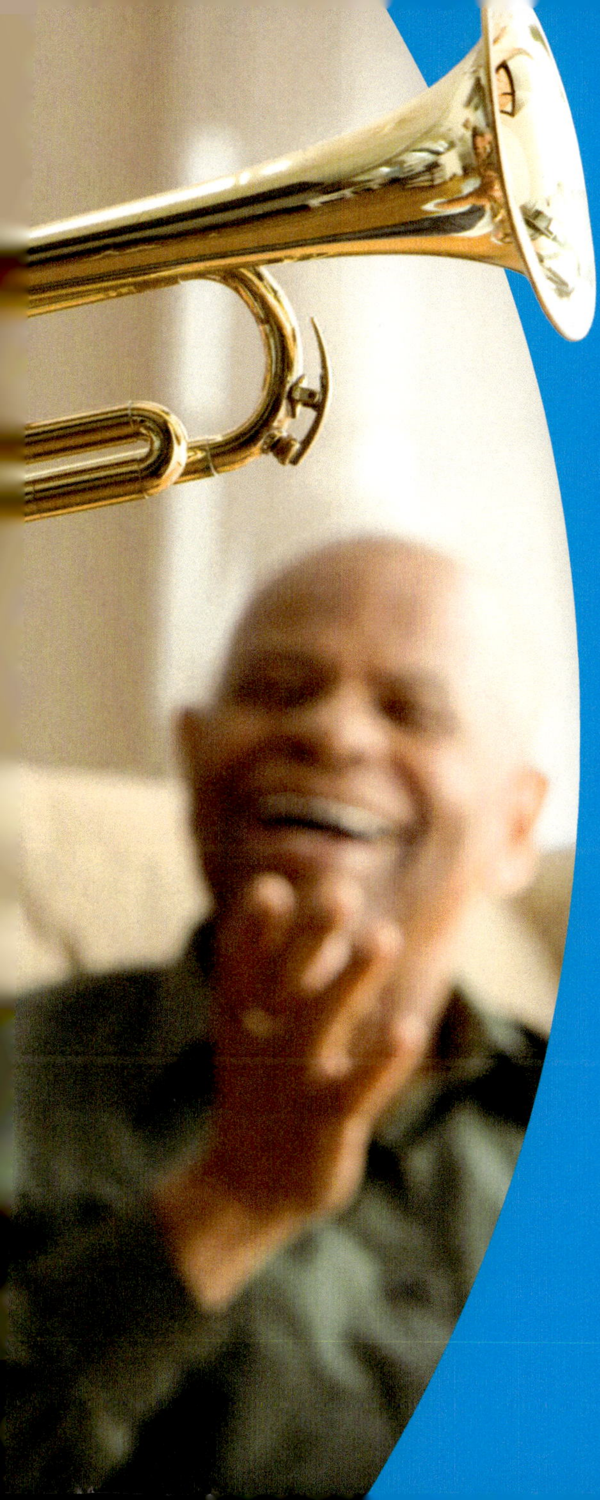

Toot! Toot!

Ben plays
the trumpet.

Which body part
do they use?

The mouth!

Look at Win's lips.
The skin is thin.
It is soft.
It is pink.

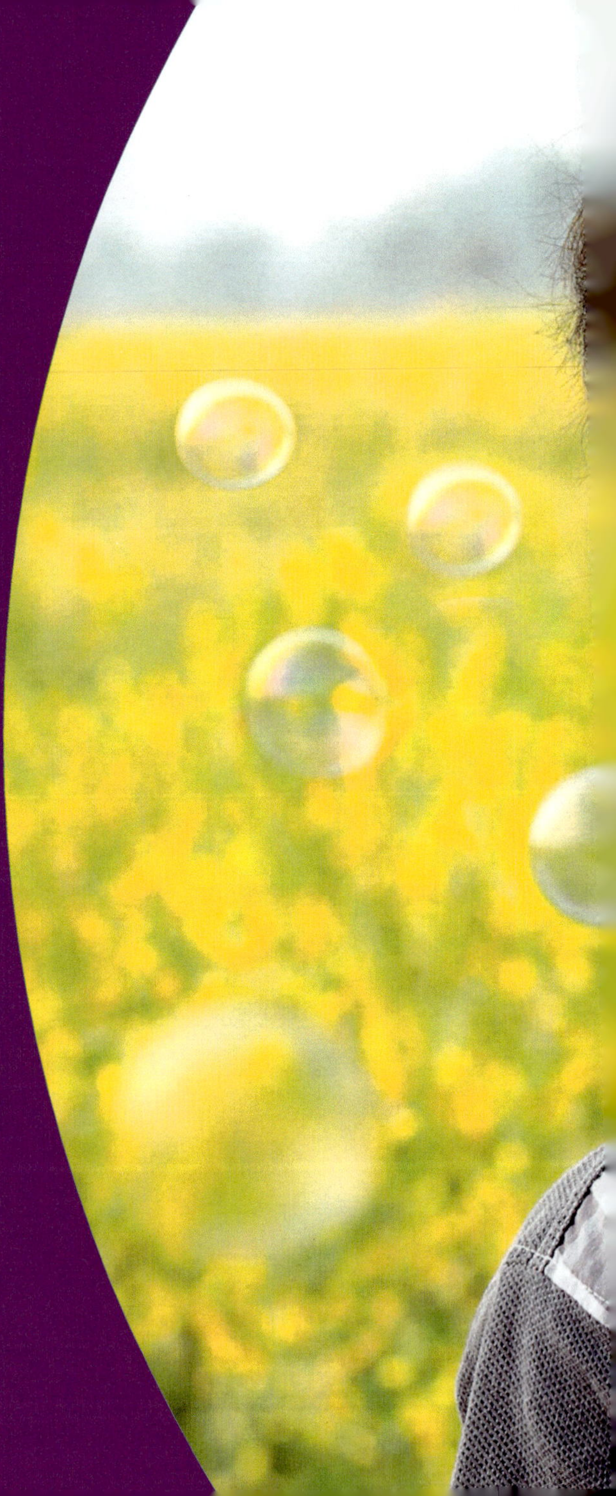

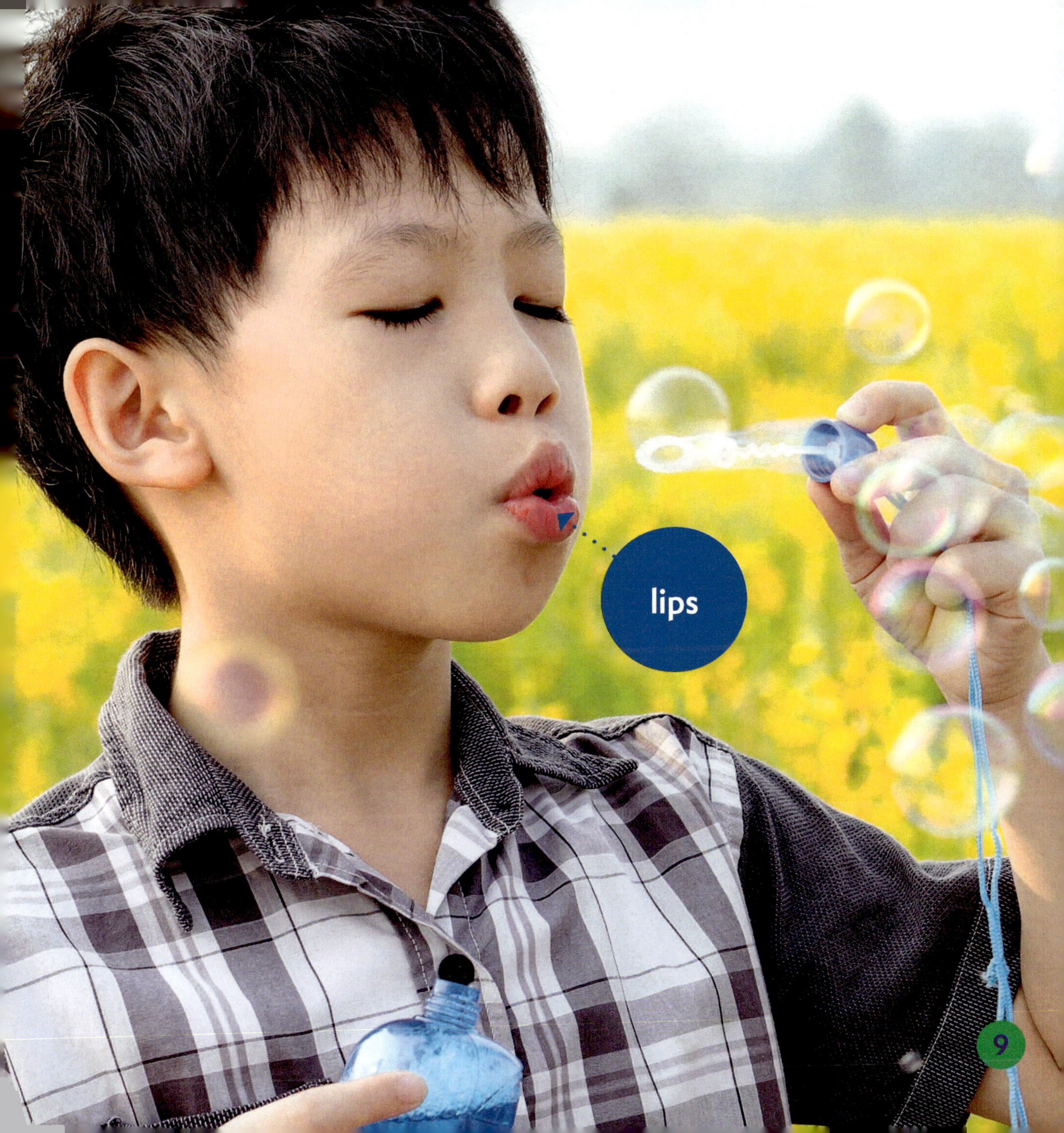
lips

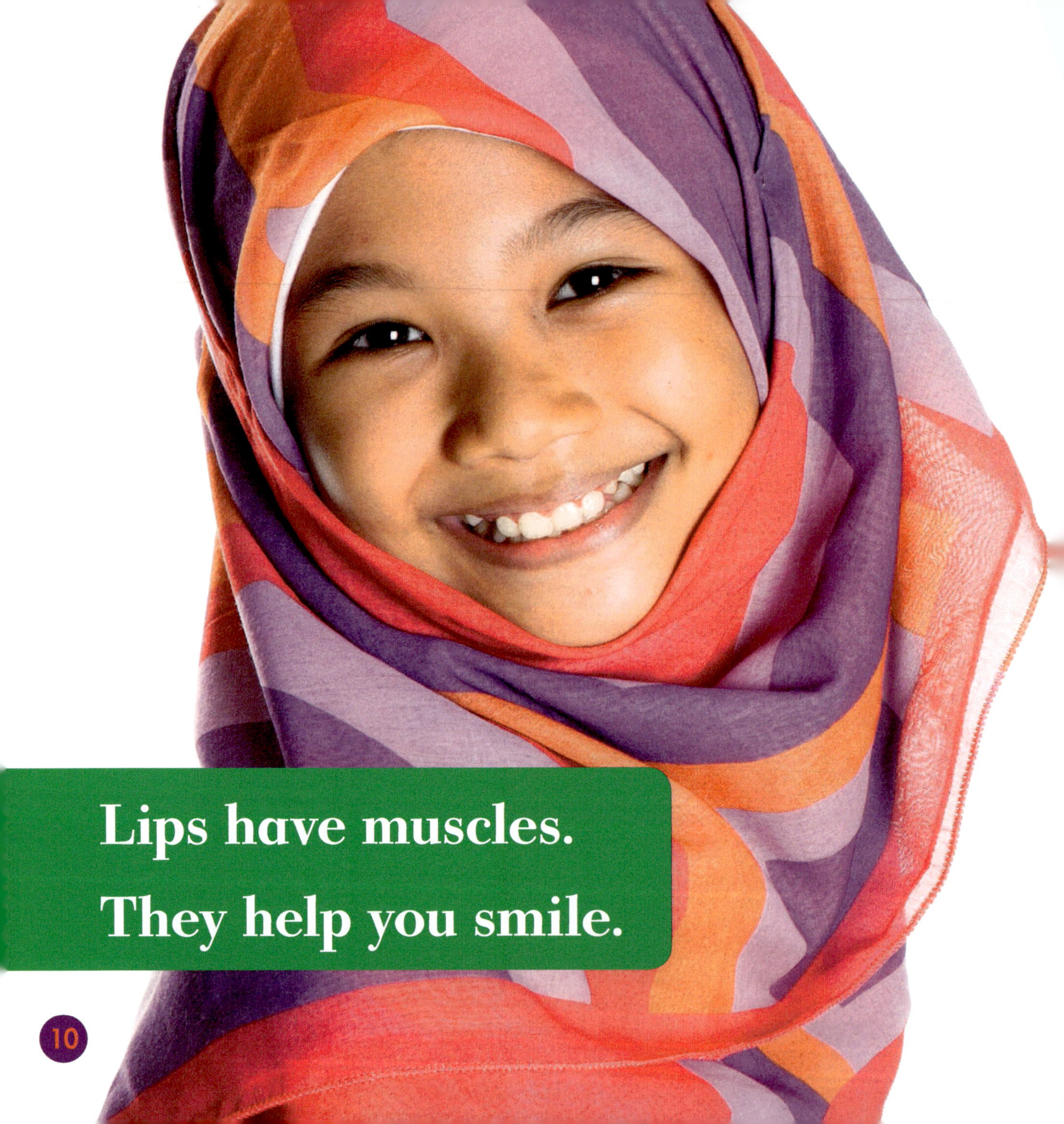

Lips have muscles.
They help you smile.

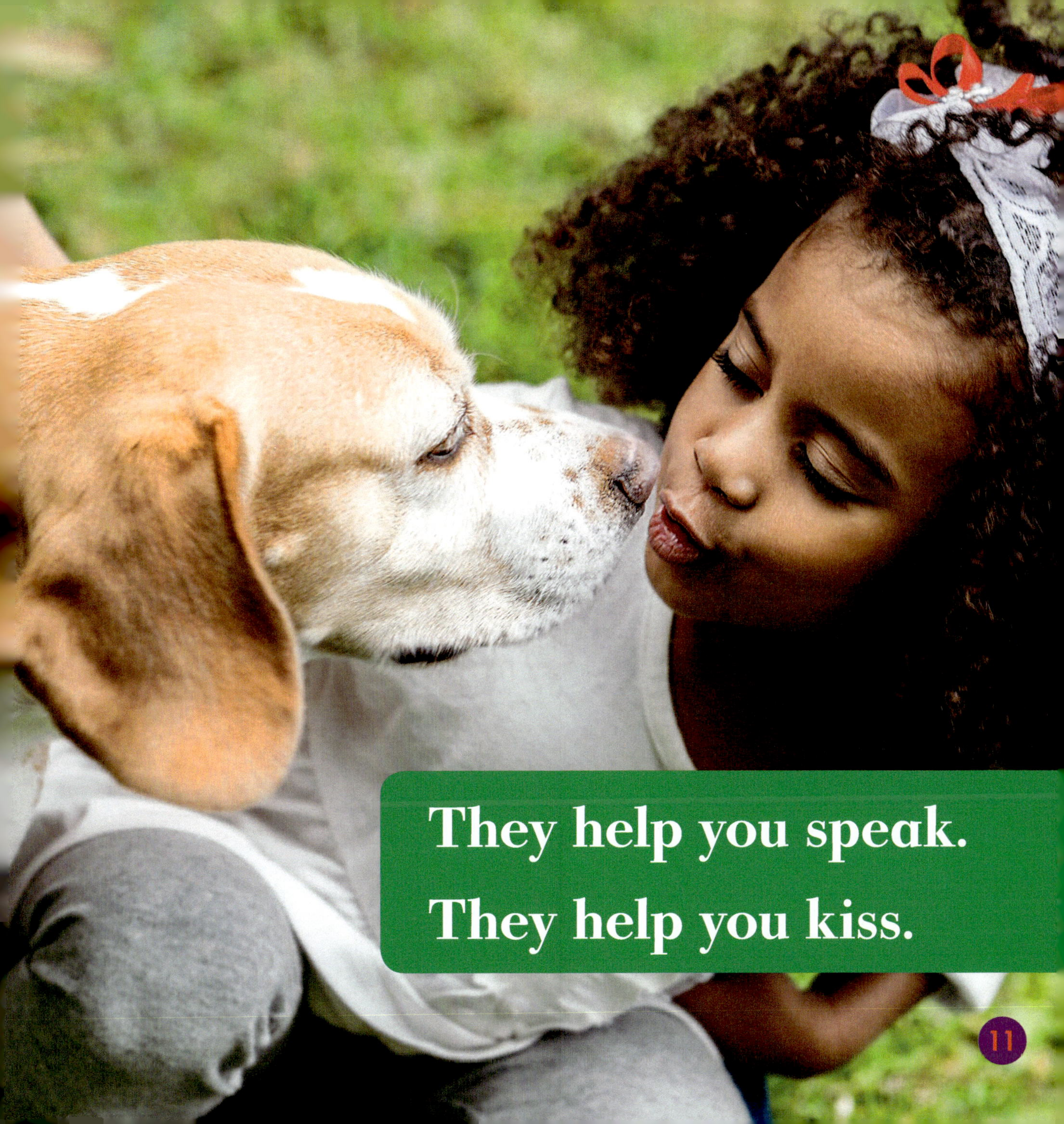

They help you speak.
They help you kiss.

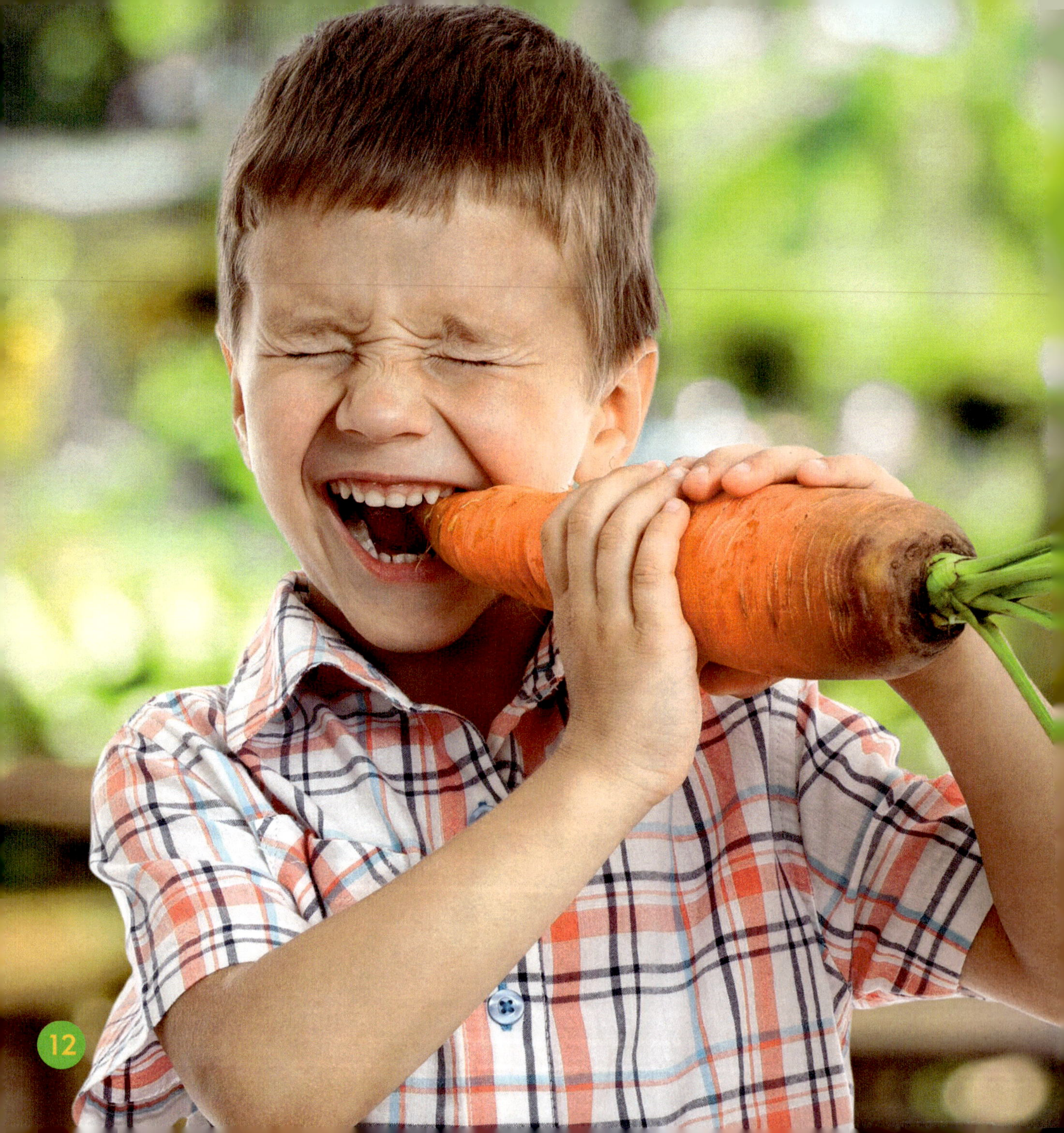

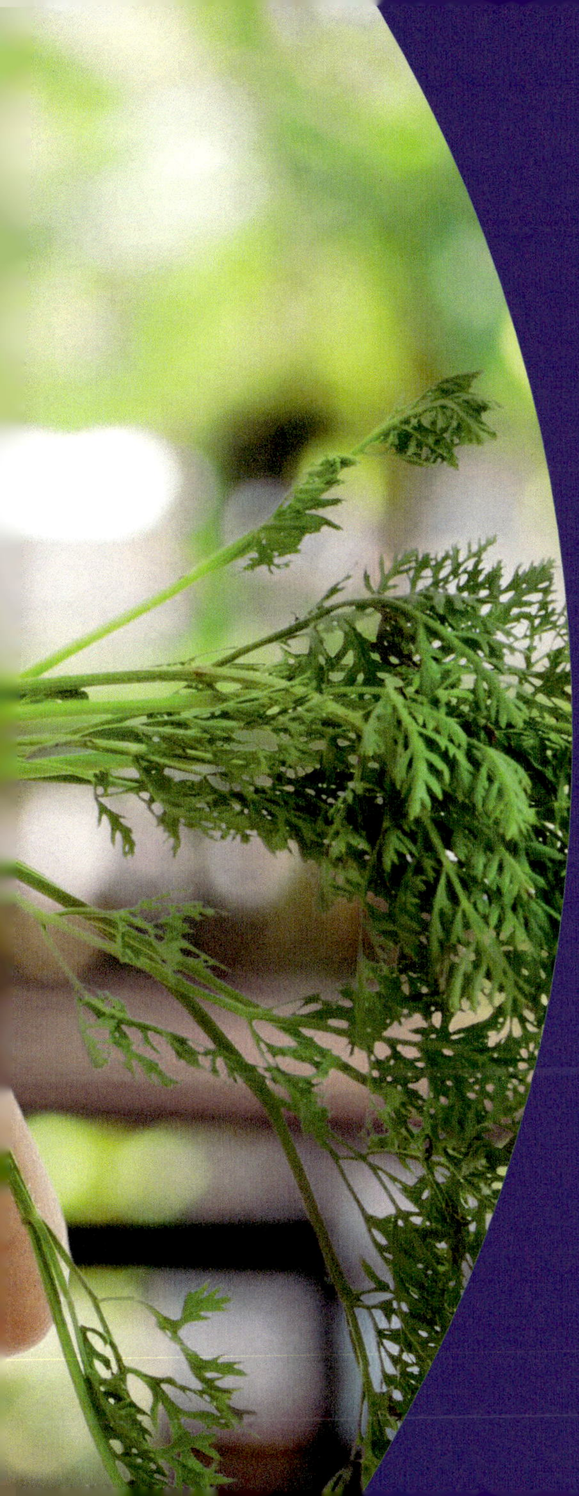

Look at Tim's teeth.

Chomp!

He bites.

He chews.

Teeth have enamel.

It is the hardest thing in the body.

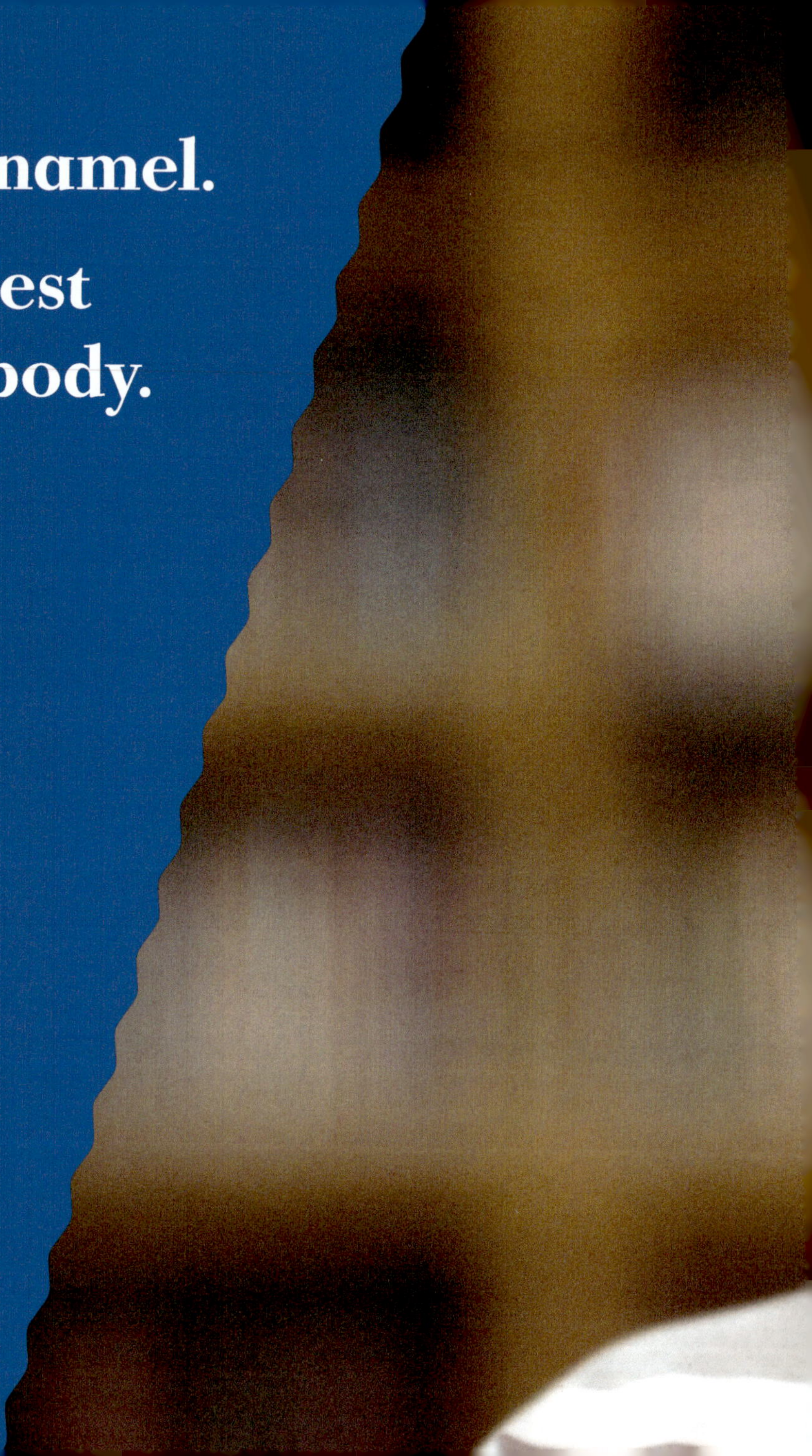

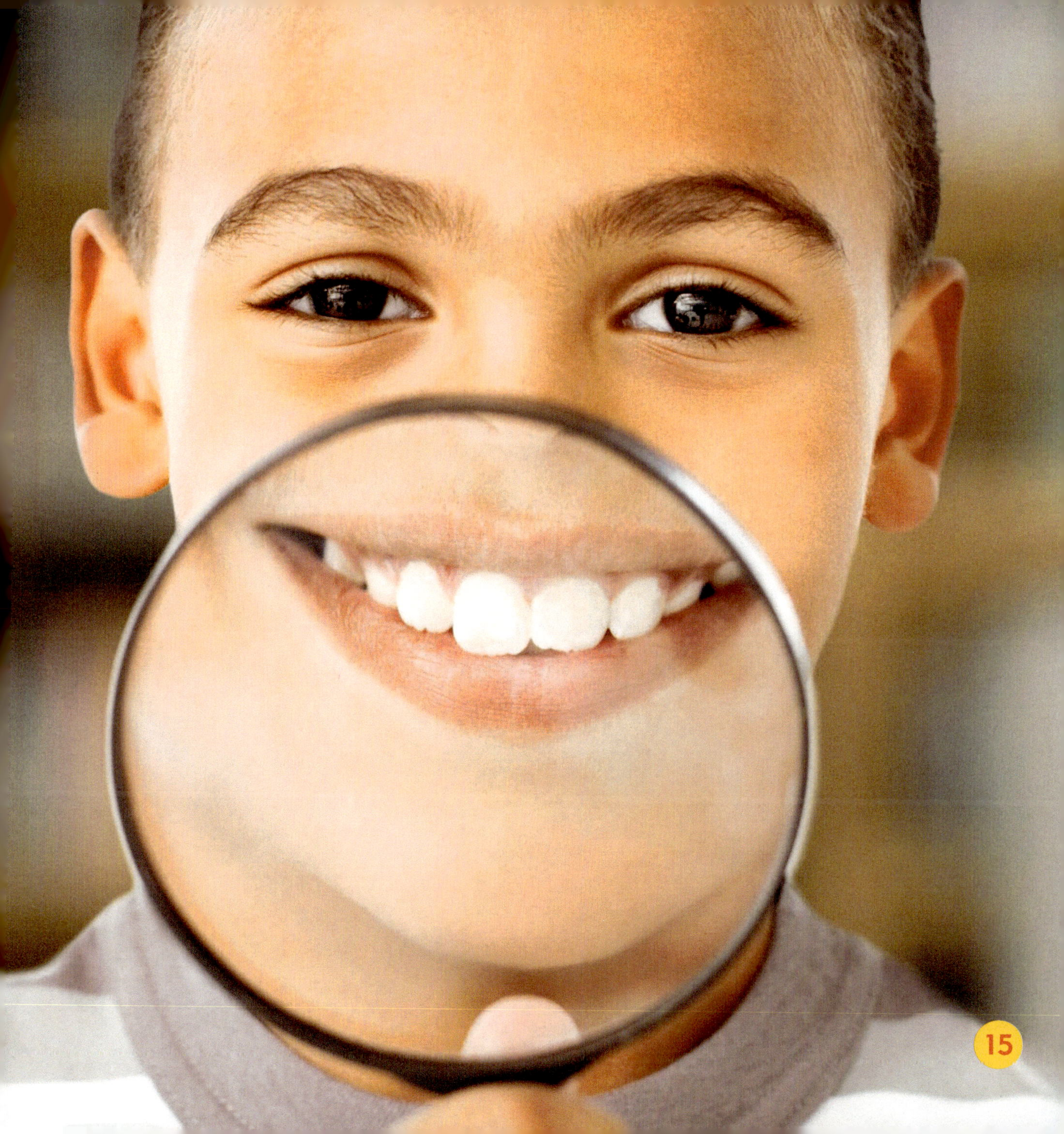

Look at Ji's tongue. It has taste buds.

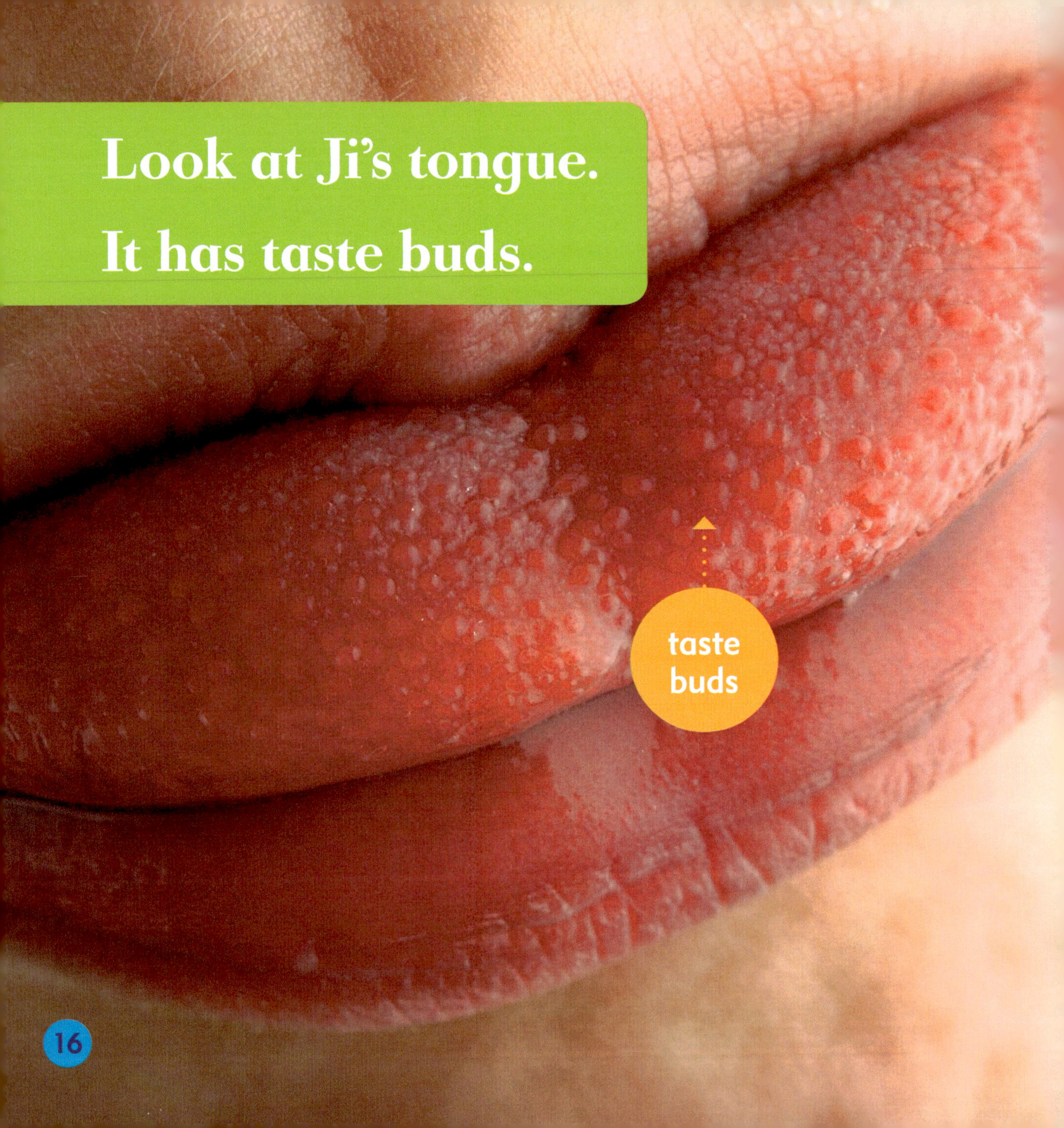

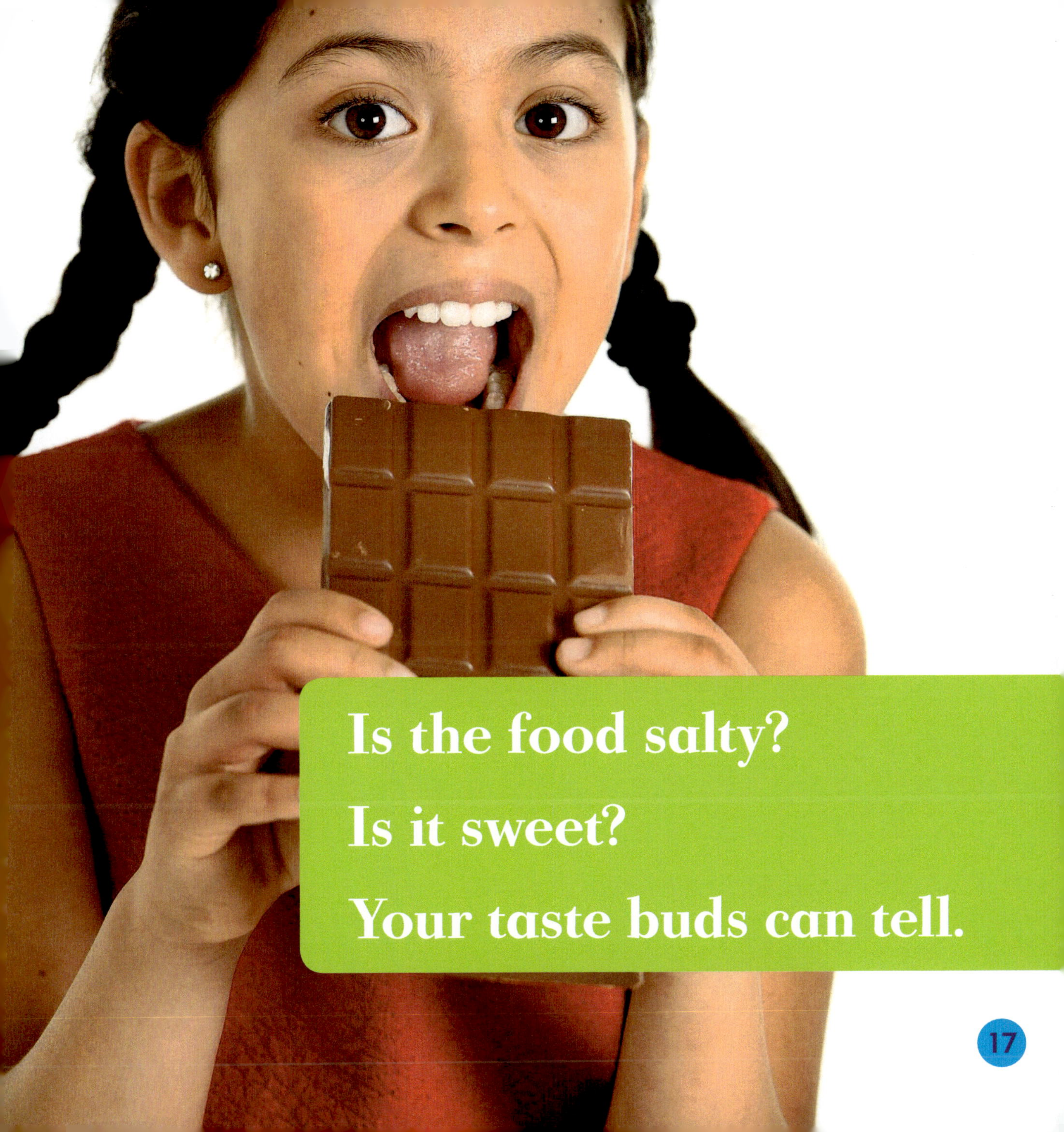

Is the food salty?

Is it sweet?

Your taste buds can tell.

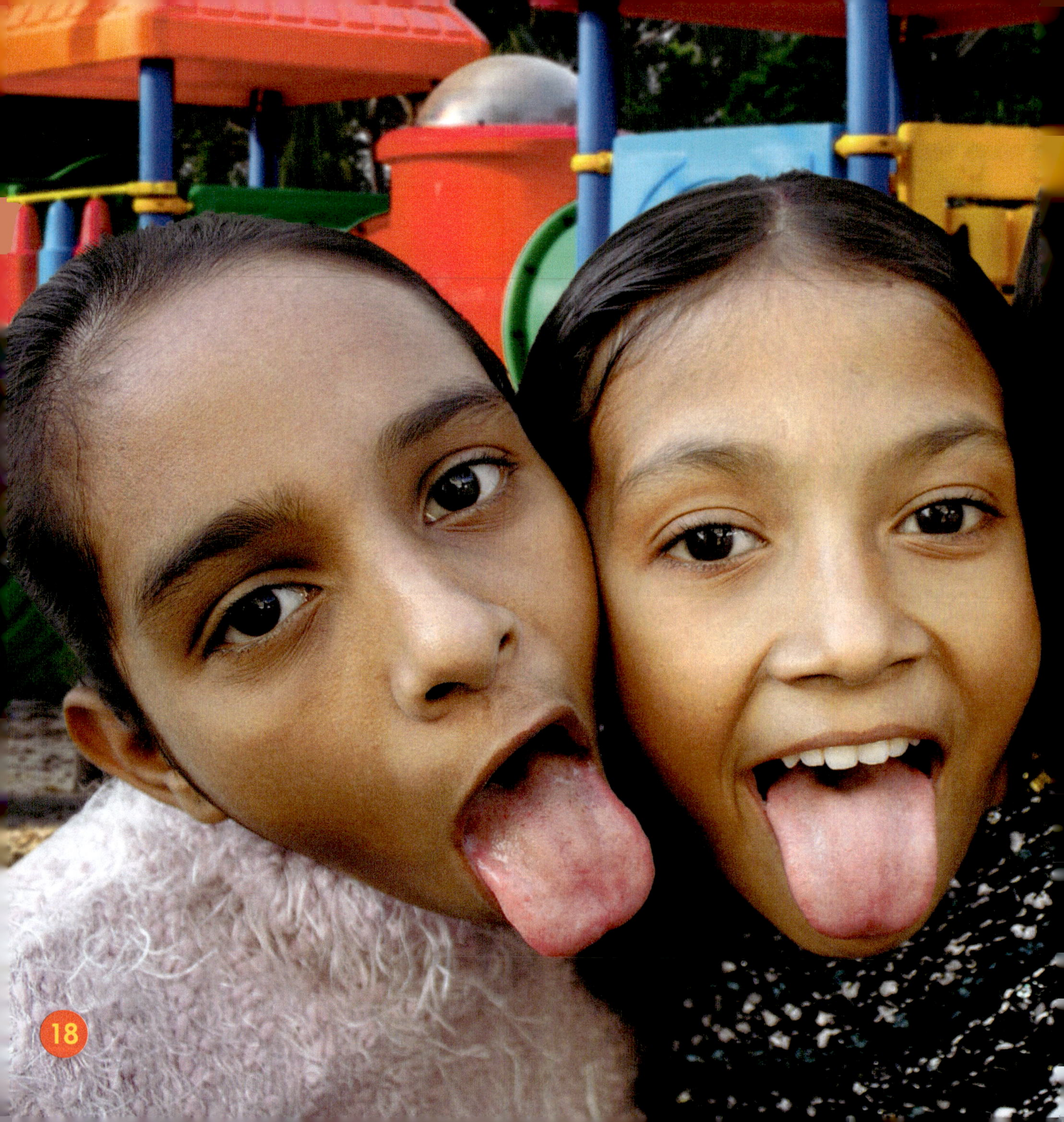

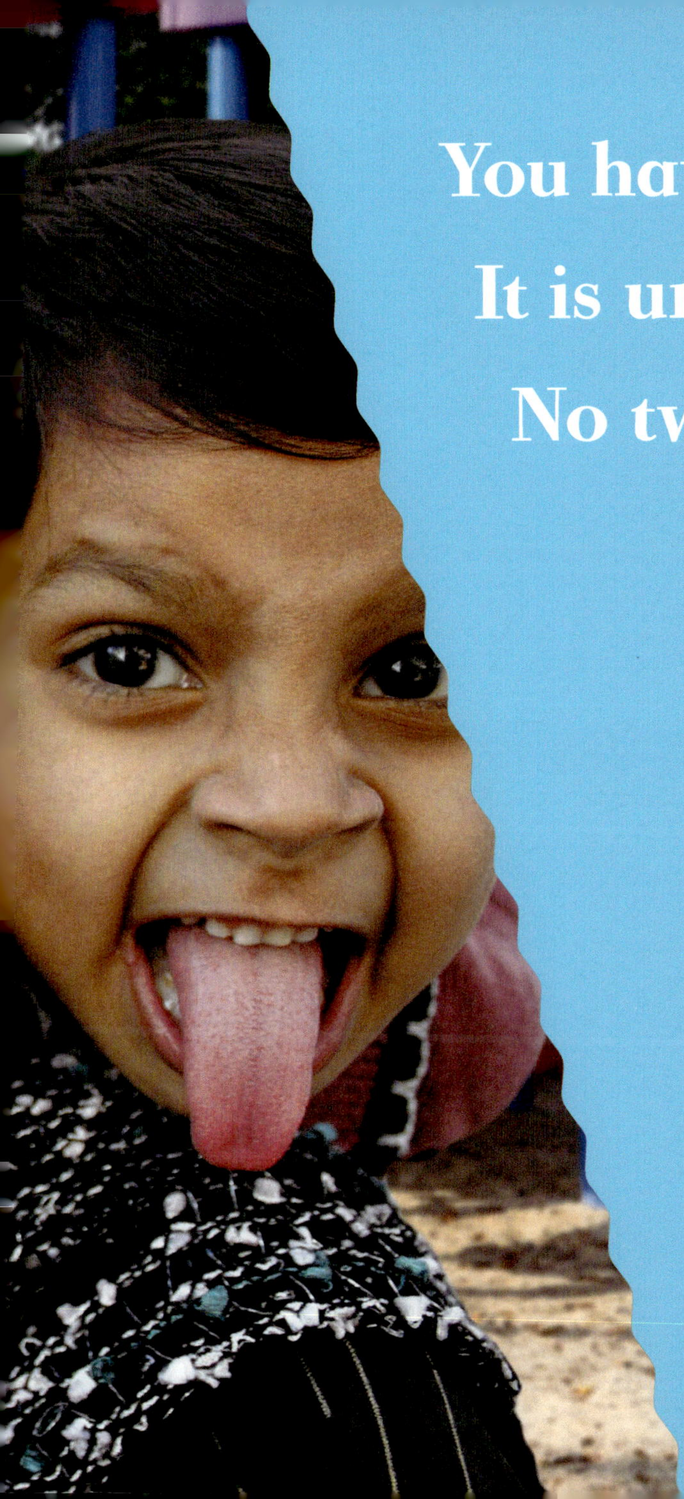

You have a tongue print.

It is unique.

No two are the same!

So smile! Talk!
Chew! Sing!

Your mouth is cool!

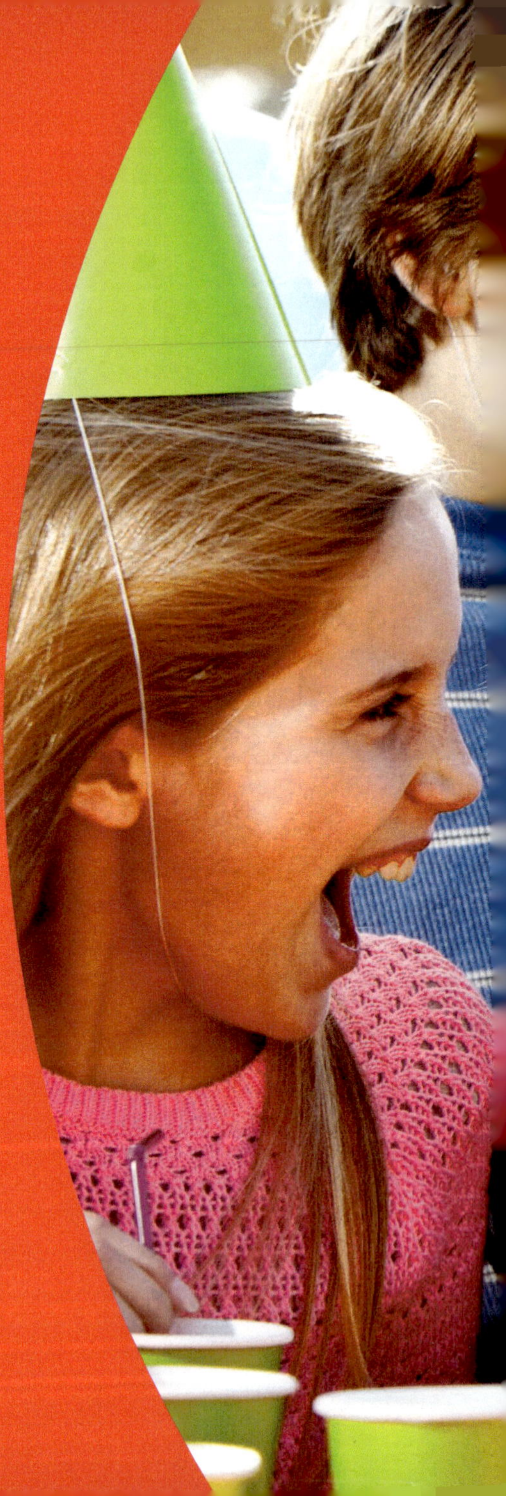

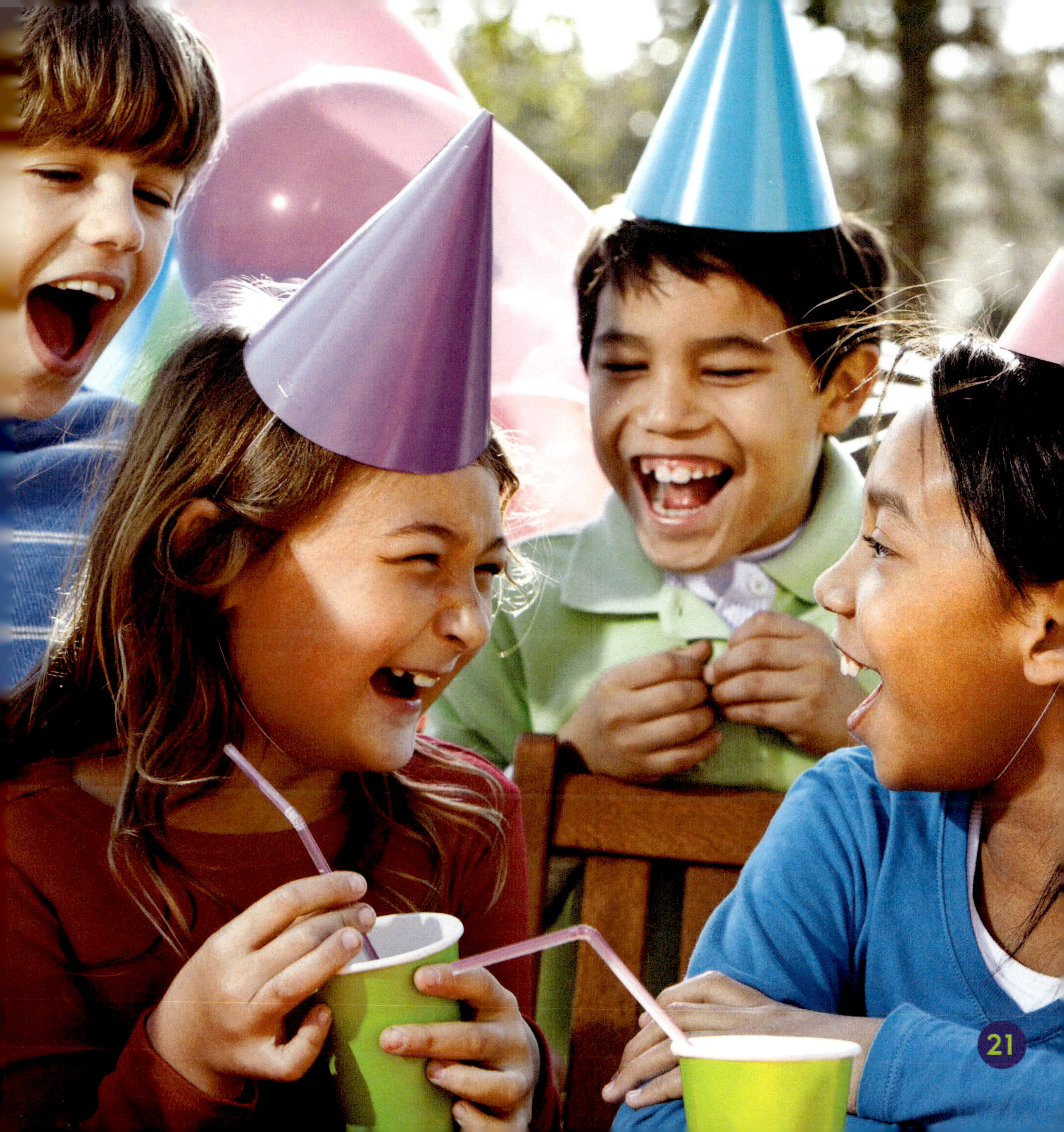

Parts of the Mouth

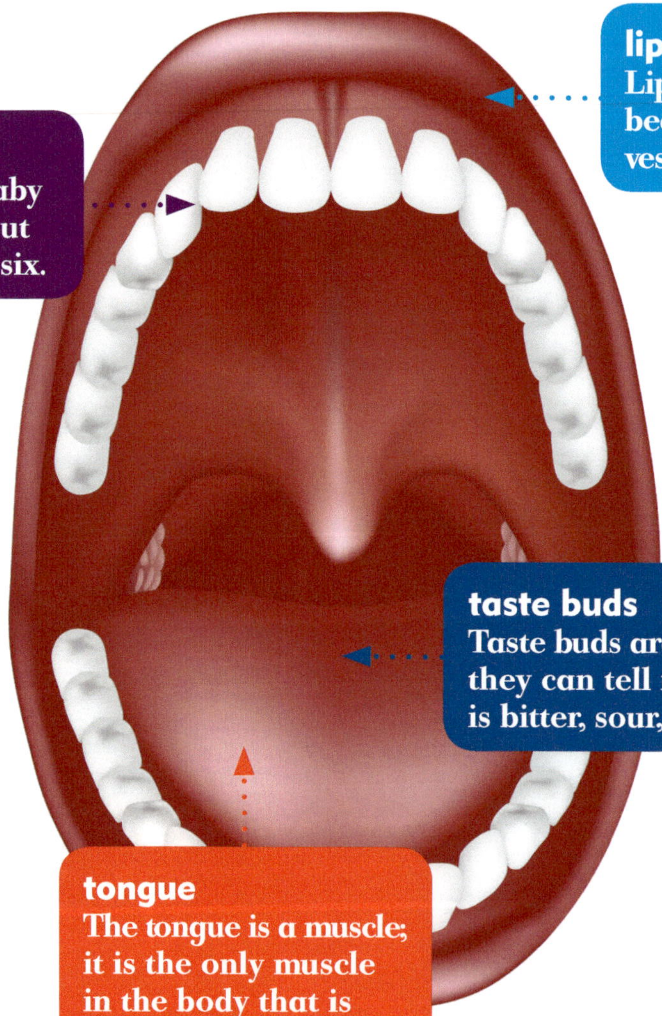

lips
Lips are pink or red because of the blood vessels underneath.

teeth
Your first baby tooth falls out around age six.

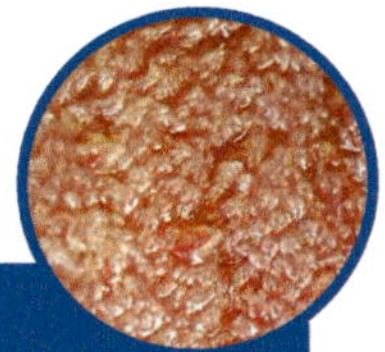

taste buds
Taste buds are nerve endings; they can tell if something is bitter, sour, salty, or sweet.

tongue
The tongue is a muscle; it is the only muscle in the body that is detached on one end.

Picture Glossary

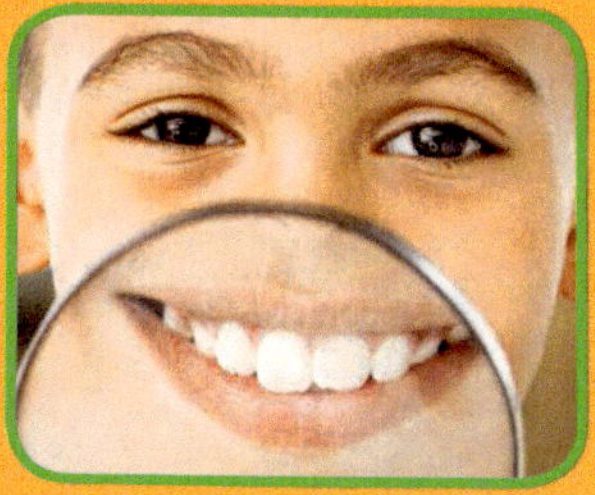

enamel
The hard, outer layer of your teeth.

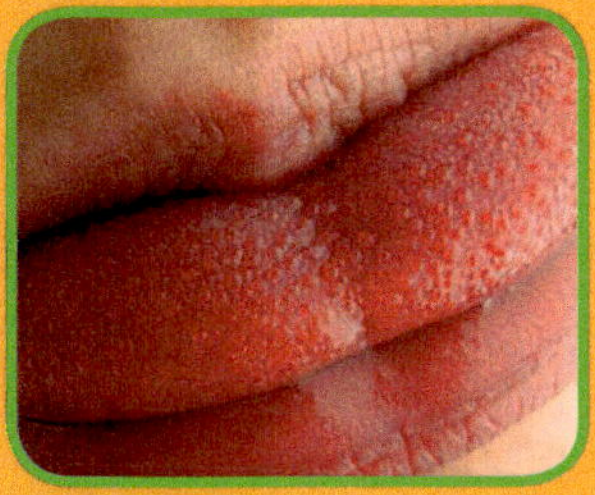

tongue print
The marks and shapes that make up someone's tongue.

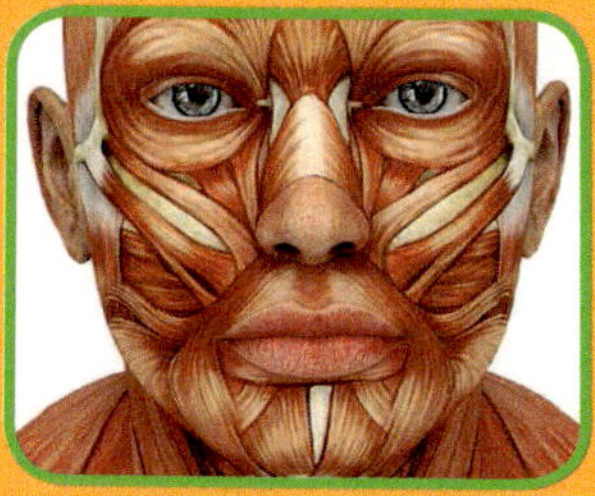

muscles
The part of your body that makes movement.

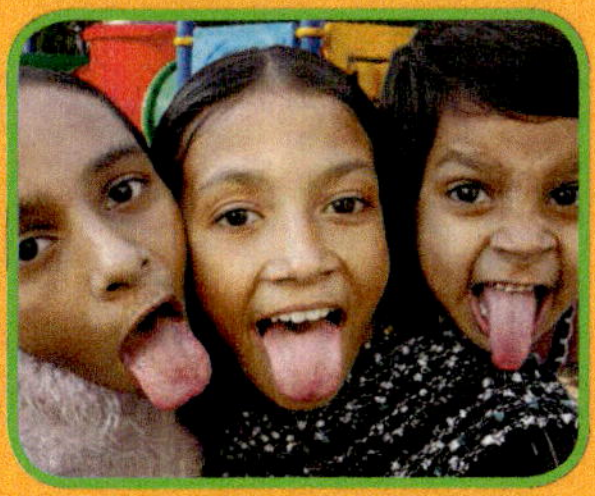

unique
One-of-a-kind, unlike any other.

Index

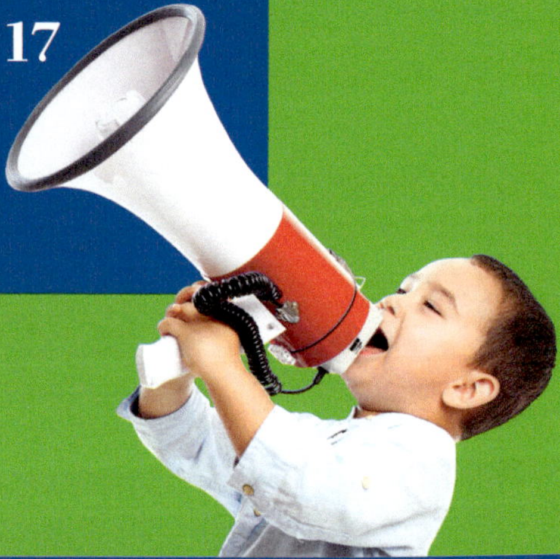

To Learn More

Learning more is as easy as 1, 2, 3.

1) Go to www.factsurfer.com
2) Enter "mouth" into the search box.
3) Click the "Surf" button to see a list of websites.

With factsurfer.com, finding more information is just a click away.